MINDSET
BREAKTHROUGH

Achieve
Weight-Loss
Surgery
Success

BETH BIANCA

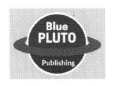

Printed in the United States of America

Mindset Breakthrough: Achieve Weight-Loss Surgery Success / Beth Bianca -- 1st ed.

ISBN-13: 978-0-692-80615-9
ISBN-10: 0-692-80615-6

Join Beth Bianca's motivational community, using your phone.
Text **LIVING** to **444999**

Meet Beth Bianca online at:
www.BethBianca.com

Digital and print formatting completed by Perry Elisabeth Design.

DEDICATION

This book is dedicated to my Mom, Lou Lou. Mom was my biggest cheerleader and believed in me when I didn't even believe in myself. Her love, encouragement, and friendship were an inspiration to everyone who knew her.

Mom, I was so blessed to have been your baby. I miss and love you more than I can ever say. I wish you were here with us now, but I know you are with me in spirit. Thank you for all the seeds you planted in my life while you were here. They are still blooming.

ACKNOWLEDGEMENTS

First and foremost, I thank God for giving me a second opportunity to live, love and grow. Thank you for giving me the opportunity to share this message of transformation and to continue forward with my life's purpose.

To my aunt, Nancy. Thank you for your love and prayers, especially during my darkest days. You always believed, even when I didn't, that I would gain my health back. You are the cornerstone that provides strength and support in my life.

To my sister, Carlene, who has been with me through all of life's ups and downs. Thank you for your support during my weakest days and for celebrating my victories. You have helped to mold me into the person I am today. You are the sunshine in my life.

To my lifelong friend, Lydia. You were there to help pick up the pieces when my life fell apart. You have been there during my darkest days and in the brightest. Your friendship, support and compassion have brought me through my bleakest hours. Thank you for always being there for me. You are my lighthouse during the storm and the glistening rays of joy in my life.

To my dear friend, Gina. Thank you for providing a vision for me when I had no sight of my future. There is a thread woven into our lives that has connected us through the twists and turns of life. We can't see the pattern being weaved, but every stitch has strengthened our friendship. You add color to the tapestry of my life.

To my fellow Bariatric Weight Warriors. Our stories may be different, but we share a similar experience. You inspire me to continue on this path. Your love for living and not merely existing is an example to all who might take life for granted. We can do this!

TABLE OF CONTENTS

Introduction   9

Chapter One: Too Much to Lose   13

Chapter Two: Knowing What to Do   19

Chapter Three: Do What You Know   29

Chapter Four: Train Your Brain   33

Chapter Five: Lights, Camera, Action   49

Chapter Six: Habitual Behaviors   57

Chapter Seven: The Secret Sauce of Success   63

Chapter Eight: The Power of Your Thoughts   69

Conclusion   75

Bibliography   81

About the Author   85

INTRODUCTION

If weight-loss surgery alone helps people lose weight, why do so many people gain their weight back? Knowing what to do and then doing it is the hardest part of adapting to a new healthy lifestyle. If you are like me, before weight-loss surgery you most likely tried many diets and exercise programs only to end up gaining the weight back, plus more.

In this book, I will show you how to align your weight-loss surgery with your habits for lasting success. There are eight steps to change your thinking. By changing how you think about food and exercise, you will finally know what true weight-loss success feels like.

I yo-yo dieted my entire adult life until I ended up weighing 394 pounds. I was riddled with health issues and was housebound, unable to walk without help. I had a Vertical Sleeve Gastrectomy in April of 2015, and I currently weigh 170 pounds. The hardest part of my journey was not the surgery; instead, it was dealing with all the old thoughts and behaviors I had about food my entire life. I'm sorry to say those old thoughts and behaviors were not removed during surgery.

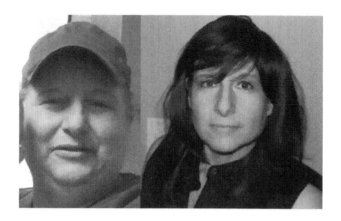

Although I had gone through the extensive pre-surgery classes and testing, I was not prepared for the mental battle that began when I arrived home after the surgery. By using the steps I describe in this book, I found the help I needed to break through my old thinking and behavior. Instead of feeling deprived, I became empowered to rebuild my life from the inside and outside.

If you follow this action plan, you will not have to worry about weight regain. When you follow these eight steps to change your thinking about food and exercise, your weight-loss surgery journey will be easier and more successful than you thought possible.

Don't be the person who waits too long to change their thinking about food and ends up dealing with head hunger, emotional eating and weight gain. Be the person who uses this "tool" of weight-loss surgery to lose their weight once and for all. Be the person who takes control of their thoughts and their body for a lifelong transformation.

The eight steps you are about to read are the same steps I used to lose 224 pounds with no long term stalls or weight gains. This works. If I could do it, so can you.

CHAPTER ONE

TOO MUCH TO LOSE

When I let go of what I am, I become what I might be.
Lao Tzu

An old adage says everyone has a burden to bear in life, and if that is true, my weight issue is mine. My life-long battle was with weight gain, weight loss and regain, plus more, over and over. I went through fad diets and exercise regimes and back to sedentary over-eating until I weighed 394 pounds.

I lost hundreds of pounds over the years and gained hundreds back, but I was always a healthy, active person through all the ups and downs. That was until February of 2011. Something changed almost overnight. I took my fur-baby (dog) out for a walk and could barely make it back to my door. Each step I took became heavier and heavier. When I finally made it to the hallway of my building, it stretched out before me, unbelievably long, like something from *The Twilight Zone*. I was completely out of breath and felt like I was going to pass out. At the time, I thought it was a onetime weird occurrence. Maybe I was getting the flu. However, that was only the beginning of a downward spiral that took over two years to be diagnosed.

Everything I did became unbearably hard. My household cleaning was the first chore to be neglected. The dishes started to pile up in the sink, the dust began to build on my furniture and there were tumble-furs in all the corners. Was I just getting lazy? It seemed like I could sleep all day long. I had absolutely no energy. After nine years of running a successful small business, I had to close it down. My inability to handle the stress became too much. Even when I took a shower, I felt like I was running a marathon. I was so out of breath I had to lean on the walls just to get through it.

I kept going to my doctor and having tests, but she could never find anything conclusive for my symptoms. I always heard the same thing: "You need to lose weight." It's not like being overweight was new to me. I had dealt with weight issues my entire life. I knew there was something more going on with the way I felt.

By October of 2013, I could barely walk out of my home. It was getting harder to keep my condition a secret. Anyone who saw me knew that something was obviously wrong. I didn't want to worry the important people in my life. But that train had left the station. At my sister's and best friend's urging, I scheduled another doctor's appointment. My sister came with me this time. My doctor ran more tests, and I was finally diagnosed with Pulmonary Hypertension.

I was so glad to finally have a name for what was causing my life to disintegrate. Yay for me! I was not crazy or lazy; I had Pulmonary Hypertension. I didn't really know what that was, so I decided to dig around on the internet to find out more. What I found out that night was nothing to celebrate. Pulmonary Hypertension occurs when arteries in the lung become damaged and can no longer move blood the way they are supposed to. There really isn't a cure, but doctors try to treat the symptoms for as long as they can. Depending on the stage at which you are diagnosed, the prognosis could be as little as one year to maybe over ten years to live.

Next, I had to figure at what stage I had just been diagnosed. That, of course, was related to how out of breath a person becomes after activity. According to that information, I was in a stage three out of four. That gave me three to five years left. My whole world came crashing down. With the way I was feeling, I didn't think I'd make it a year. Month by month, my breathing was getting worse. There was a noticeable difference to the daily activities I could complete.

My Pulmonary Hypertension had been caused by sleep apnea. I didn't even know I had sleep apnea, but apparently it had been a part of my life for so long it became severe enough to damage the arteries in my lungs. After a sleep study, I was also diagnosed with both obstructive and central sleep apnea. Another "goody" for me. Instead of having a CPAP machine, which provides constant air pressure, I was prescribed a BiPAP machine. The BiPAP machine provides air pressure when I inhale and stops when I exhale. The providers told me it works like a ventilator. How wonderful was that? It was just another reason to expect the worst case scenario. Besides that, I also had developed Type II Diabetes, a fatty liver, high blood pressure and three herniated discs in my back.

My doctor said losing weight would help to relieve a lot of my symptoms. She brought up having weight-loss surgery. However, we had to stabilize my health issues first. I prepared for the worst. I didn't want to leave a mess behind after I died.

Eventually, I made it to the weight-loss surgery seminar. All the while my breathing kept getting worse. Between the seminar and the first consultation appointment, I had to start using a wheelchair. Between the first consultation and my surgery day, I couldn't leave my home. I was unable to do anything by that point. My sister and best friend took care of everything for me. My sister came and took my fur-baby for walks. They did my grocery shopping and house cleaning. Every little thing a healthy person takes for granted became impossible for me to do. I was incapacitated and was ready to die. I wasn't living, and I didn't even know if that was considered surviving.

Finally, my big day arrived in April of 2015. Surgery day was a new birthday, the day I was given a second chance at life.

I've had wonderful success with my journey. I lost a total of 224 pounds and gained my life back. I can once again do all the things most people take for granted, and no wheelchair, walker or cane is needed for walking. But I will never forget how it was during those dark days.

I am no longer on any Diabetes medications. My blood pressure and liver functions are normal. I still use a BiPAP machine when I sleep, but the pressure has been reduced dramatically. I'm not sure if I will ever be able to stop using it completely, but I am totally fine with that either way. I actually enjoy breathing while I sleep. Go figure. As for the Pulmonary Hypertension, most of the time I don't even realize it's there. It is harder to breathe on high humidity days, so I just make sure to stay in air conditioned areas.

The most important change is that I no longer feel like I'm slowly dying. According to the same chart I read after my diagnosis, I'm back down to a stage one. My doctors say that Pulmonary Hypertension shouldn't hinder me from living a full life as long as I keep my weight stable and continue to monitor my sleep apnea. Plus, new ways of dealing with Pulmonary Hypertension are being discovered every year. All in all, I'm a whole new person. I feel alive and have hope for my future again.

Weight-loss surgery is certainly not the easy way to lose weight. I believe, like many others, that the surgery is a tool which gives us an opportunity to finally lose weight. I suffered through a lifetime of weight-loss failures, but this time, with the right tool and the knowledge of how to use it properly, I was able to accomplish what seemed impossible.

What some people don't understand is that weight-loss surgery only works when we change our thoughts and behaviors about food. It's not a magic pill, and there is no secret formula. The process takes commitment, dedication and perseverance to reach and maintain our goals, but I thank God every day for giving me this second opportunity to learn, live and fulfill my purpose in life.

There you have Step 1: Know Your Story. We must accept the past for what it was. However, we cannot allow the past to define our future. Now you know a little about me. Let's get started with Step 2: The Bariatric Basics, which I used to change my life.

CHAPTER TWO

KNOWING WHAT TO DO

You are going to be successful because you are going to do two things.
You're going to learn new things, and then you are going to do them.
T. Harv Eker

There are two ingredients to a successful weight-loss surgery journey. First, you need to know the "Bariatric Basics." Second, you need to use them consistently for the rest of your life. But don't get too frightened by that. The steps found in the following chapters will give you the system needed to apply what you learn through a proven process that works.

As we begin with Step 2: The Bariatric Basics, I want to stress the importance of following the specific instructions given to you by your surgeon. What I am sharing with you are the Bariatric Basics that have worked for me. They were the instructions provided to me during my nutrition classes, which were taught by my bariatric surgery team at a Center of Excellence facility. This has been my blueprint for consistent weight-loss success. If you have gone through nutrition classes, this is intended to be a refresher for you. It is not meant to replace the instructions provided by your surgery team.

1 - Keep a Food Journal — You must know exactly what you are eating and how often. Every item you eat needs to be logged, including snacks. Total calories for the day should be no more or less than your doctor recommends for your post-op stage. Sometimes keeping a food journal is the first thing people stop doing. I plan on using a food journal for the rest of my life. When you log your food, there is no way for weight-gain to sneak up on you. You can track your food by using online apps like Baritastic and Myfitnesspal.com or just keep a simple paper and pen journal. Pick something easy to use. The most important part of picking the right food journal is to find one you will actually use.

2 - Breakfast — *Eat something the first 30 minutes after waking up.* In the article titled, "The Half-Hour Window," at RiversideOnline.com" [Ref-1], they explain that when we are sleeping at night our body shifts into a fat storing mode to conserve energy while we sleep. They go on to state, "Eating a meal within 30 minutes of waking will help increase the rate of our metabolism which has slowed down to conserve the stored energy." The article continues, "The longer you wait to eat, the greater the risk your metabolism will slow down and shift into the fat-storing starvation mode." This seems like a pretty simple step to start the day off strong. There is no reason for my metabolism to be sleeping when I have already started my day. Sometimes I have a low-fat cheese stick within 15 minutes of waking up. Then I have my full breakfast an hour later when I have more time.

3 - Protein — Needs vary depending on your post-op stage. According to the UCLA's Bariatric Program Material [Ref – 2] they recommend between 60-90 grams of protein per day. Make sure you do what it takes to meet your protein requirements every day.

4 - Water — Drink 64 oz per day. This includes the water you mix with protein powder and/or use in decaffeinated tea. After weight-loss surgery, because the size of our stomach has been reduced, it is more difficult for us to get our necessary water intake. We need to be especially careful not to become dehydrated. When consuming beverages, we should avoid caffeine and carbonated drinks. In the Johns Hopkins [Ref-3] bariatric information guide, they explain why: "Carbonation may cause abdominal discomfort and may stretch out your new stomach over time. Caffeine may irritate the stomach and increase your risk for an ulcer after surgery." Another important item to mention is that you should drink all beverages between meals, not during the meal. In an article from the Bariatric Surgery Source [Ref-4] they state, "You can't drink with your meals and need to wait at least an hour after you eat before drinking anything. If you don't, the liquids will quickly flush the food through your stomach. This can affect digestion, make you feel hungry and lead to weight gain after bariatric surgery."

5 - Vitamins — Always take your doctor's recommended dosage of vitamins. This is another way to avoid malnutrition and is extremely important for bariatric patients.

6 - Exercise — Get plenty of exercise. The American Heart Association [Ref-5] recommends, "At least 30 minutes of moderate-intensity aerobic activity at least 5 days per week for a total of 150" minutes per week. I have to admit, since I wasn't even able to walk at the time of my surgery, this is a goal that took some time to reach. Find what exercise works best for you and gradually build your endurance. Any type of exercise is better than none.

7 - Avoid temptation — Don't even try one of your impulse foods or beverages. Once you open that door, it is hard to close it again. It's definitely not worth the damage that may result from a little indulgence.

I use the following information as my guideline when preparing meals. It helps me to make a good per serving food choice. It was provided to me by my nutritionist and it has worked great.

- Protein - 10 grams or higher (the higher it is the better)
- Fat - 5 grams or less
- Sugar - 5 grams or less (only exception is skim milk)

WEIGHT-LOSS STALLS

The Scale Isn't Always Your Friend. After my Vertical Sleeve Gastrectomy surgery, I hit a plateau during week six. At this point I had already lost a total of 87 pounds, with only 30 of that being post-surgery. I didn't even think it was possible to have a stall so soon after surgery. I emailed my nutritionist to see if this was normal. She said that it definitely was normal and that, once my body was over it, I would see a jump in lost pounds. She raised my protein up to 88 grams per day. The next week I lost 3.5 pounds.

First and foremost, DO NOT let a scale plateau ever take you off track. Everyone who has ever lost weight has hit a stall at some point. If you have a lot of weight to lose, you will most likely hit more than one stall.

An article at ObesityCoverage.com [Ref-6] describes a plateau as this:

> Your body is constantly seeking something called homeostasis. Homeostasis is a process that maintains the human body's internal environment in response to changes in external conditions. So when food decreases significantly (external condition), your body adjusts internally to create stability (stable weight). So, to counteract the lack of food in your environment, the body slows down your basal metabolic rate – your metabolism slows down and

you hit a wall. You haven't changed your eating or exercise habits and you hit a wall before you reach your target weight.

In other words, in order to have hit a plateau, you have already lost some weight. Pause to reflect on the progress you have already made. Plateaus are like going through puberty: It just happens. We may not enjoy it, but we can get through it, and sometimes we can get through it with style. The following paragraphs will give you some ways of dealing with that dreaded plateau.

MUSCLE VS. FAT

An article in Everydayhealth.com [Ref-7] provides a great description of the difference between muscle and fat: "Common sense tells us a pound of muscle and a pound of fat have to weigh the same, but they do differ in density. This means if you look at five pounds of muscle and five pounds of fat side by side, the fat takes up more volume, or space, than the muscle." Because of this, when we strengthen our muscle through exercise, we will lose fat and inches. You are actually becoming thinner and more fit. Even though the scale may not reflect the fat loss, your body composition is changing for the better. This would be reflected in your measurements, photos, and the way your clothes fit. This is what people refer to as weight redistribution. There are a number of methods to track your progress. Using the scale is only one of them.

OTHER WAYS TO TRACK FAT LOSS

Take your measurements every two weeks. Make sure you measure the same exact areas at the same time of day. You can measure your neck, pecks for the men, bust and bra line for the women, the waist (at the belly button), the largest part of your hips, your biceps and your thighs.

Take photos every three to four weeks. Make sure you take them at the same time of day and in the same type of lighting. You can even wear the same clothing if you want to see how different the clothes appear on you.

Keep a journal of all the activities you can do now that were difficult or impossible to do before. You can add to it whenever you notice a difference in something. It's a great way to remind yourself of the progress you have made.

Measure your body fat percentage weekly. Depending on how much you like gadgets, there are scales and electronic devices that will measure this. FYI, I found that using calipers is a pretty hard method to use. It is difficult to be consistent with its measurements.

Save a set of your largest clothes. It's a great motivation boost to put those old, big jeans back on and see how much smaller you are in them.

MIX IT UP

If you have been following the "Bariatric Basics" and have not shown a loss on the scale or with a reduction in measurements, here are few things you can incorporate into your routine to help kick-start your progress again.

Exercise: If you are currently walking 30 minutes per day, it's time to add some variety. Track how many steps you have been walking in 30 minutes and increase that amount by either adding more time or increasing the intensity of your walk.

Strength Training: You don't need to be a body builder, but you definitely should be toning your muscles. You can switch one of your walking days for strength training or just add it to a different time of the day. Work out with free-weights, exercise bands or your body weight to strengthen your muscles. Remember that muscle burns fat. Even if you don't see it on the scale immediately, you will in your measurements. Start by adding this one to two days per week.

Carbohydrates: Start tracking how many carbs you are eating per day. Carbohydrates turn into sugar, so this can be a hidden detriment to fat loss. The American Society for Metabolic and Bariatric Surgery (ASMBS) [Ref-8] recommends, "Limiting carbohydrates to 50 grams per day or less helps avoid rebound hunger problems which can lead to weight regain."

Accountability Partner: Working with an accountability partner is fun and encouraging. Knowing you are not alone helps to keep you on track and to stay motivated. This can be with a friend, or you can hire a professional coach.

Now you know What to Do. With Step 3 in the next chapter, we will begin to transform your thinking so that Doing What You Know comes easily and naturally for you.

CHAPTER THREE

DO WHAT YOU KNOW

You must learn a new way to think
before you can master a new way to be.
Marianne Williamson

Now that you Know What to Do, it is time for Step 3: Do What You Know. If you are anything like I was, you probably came into your weight-loss surgery journey with a lifetime of old habits. I'm depressed – I need a pizza. It's time to celebrate – Let's get a pizza. I'm bored – I'll get a pizza. These old habits were not removed with surgery. How nice would that have been? So now it is up to us to figure out how to make this new lifestyle work.

After I came home from having my Sleeve Surgery, I was not prepared for what happened. I knew exactly what and how much I could eat, or should I say sip, at that point. I had everything prepared for my recuperation, but then I was sitting in my chair, watching TV and a commercial came on for a restaurant serving all you can eat "something." It could have been anything. It was just the idea of "all you can eat." My mouth dropped, my head began to spin and I just wanted to cry. How could I be so utterly unprepared for the mental anguish? Although I had gone through six months of nutrition classes, medical tests, and a psychological evaluation, none of this had been mentioned in any of the classes or appointments.

It was disturbing for me to see the old "yo-yo dieting" mindset starting to develop in my thinking. I was feeling deprived. All I thought about was what I wanted to eat and how much of it I wanted to have. Yet I knew all the while I thought about that I couldn't indulge in any of it. My thoughts were torturing me. That was until the morning I woke up and took control of the way I was looking at food. A light bulb went off, and I finally understood how to make this work.

I remembered a seminar I had taken years ago from Bob Proctor. He used an image of a "stick person" to explain how the mind works, which was originally created by Dr. Thurman Fleet.

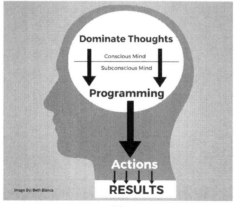

The preceding image is my interpretation of what I learned from Bob Proctor's teaching. All the results we see in our life begin with the thoughts we think. The top portion of the diagram shows the Conscious Mind above the Subconscious Mind. What we think in our conscious mind flows down into the Subconscious Mind, and then the Subconscious Mind uses those thoughts to make us perform a specific behavior. That behavior will then create the results we see in our life. Therefore, what we constantly think about becomes our reality.

Every time a behavior is performed, it creates a pathway that leads to developing a habit. Before you realize it, you don't even need to think about that behavior anymore because you just do it naturally. It has become part of your normal routine. Can you see how this worked in developing the unhealthy habits in your life?

When I think back about how a certain behavior developed, I can pinpoint when it became a habit. When I worked in an office, someone was always bringing cake or doughnuts to the lunch room. When I was first exposed to this lovely scene, I would say, "No, thank you," and continue on my merry way. But the next time I said, "Okay, just a small piece." Then the next time I just said okay. Then the next time I took a full sized piece. And, going forward from there on, my habit was to just help myself to the treats whenever they appeared.

The problem is, most of the time we do not set this program intentionally. Your subconscious does not have a reasoning ability. It guides you in the direction of what you are thinking about the most, whether that is good or bad. Sound familiar? Even though you know it is not in your best interest to eat a pizza, you still find yourself getting a pizza. Without a conscious program set, the subconscious mind uses your dominant thoughts as its programming.

Whenever you feel like you are fighting yourself, your subconscious mind trying to keep you on track with its programming, which is comprised of your old negative habits. Until you train your subconscious to know that the new behavior is more important to you, it will continue to push you toward the old behaviors. Using willpower to make a change only works for a short time before the subconscious brings you back to the old behavior.

We have to fundamentally change the program in our mind so we can build a new healthy life. We have been given a second chance to change everything, but if we use the same old program we have always used, things will eventually end up looking the same way they always did.

By changing the way you think and behave with food, you will become empowered. Instead of fighting the old habits, you will begin to build new healthy habits. You will learn how to start training your subconscious mind to work with you on your new journey, not against you. Are you ready to get started? Let's begin with Step 4: Train Your Brain.

CHAPTER FOUR

TRAIN YOUR BRAIN

Visualize this thing that you want,
See it, feel it, believe in it.
Make your mental blue print,
And begin to build.
Robert Collier

So now you know something about how your mind works. Let's get started with Step 4 and begin programming your mind to intentionally accomplish the goals you have for yourself.

After a lifetime of being overweight, my mind was programmed with habitual behaviors that were not in line with my new healthy goals. Weighing 394 pounds had wreaked havoc on my mental mindset. I had failed at so many diets that I lost count and finally gave up hope of ever losing the weight. Those failures weighed heavily on mind and body. How in the world could I change that mental programming to accomplish my big goal of being healthy and fit?

For most of our lives, our mind has been programmed by everything we have been told by our family and friends, what we see in our environments and what we personally experience. It is incredible how our brain develops during the first five years of our lives. An article written by Dr. Bill Frist entitled "Child's First 5 Years Hold Key to Success" [Ref-9] states, "Between birth and 5 years old, 90 percent of a child's brain development occurs, and at a lightning-fast pace. Every sight, smell, sound and sensation makes an impact. Long before most children step foot into a classroom, neurons are building networks, cognition is exploding, language is developing, and the foundations are being laid for a lifetime of learning." Our young brains are like sponges that soak up everything they come into contact with. There is no filter to determine if what it is being accepted is true, false, good or bad. These "stories" end up being the programs that we live with for the rest of our lives unless at some point we make a conscious decision to change the programming ourselves.

Unless you were surrounded by super high achievers and received constant positive messages from your environment, you most likely have experienced life through your emotions. When things went well, you felt great. When things were not so good, you felt bad. It's a lot like being a boat on the water without a rudder. It gets pulled back and forth by the waves and the currents, with no control of getting to its destination. Sometimes it's on top of a wave, and sometimes it drops in-between the waves.

When you are struggling in waves of emotion, life feels out of control. To start taking back that control, you need to recognize how this pattern has worked in your life. By becoming aware of the pattern, you will be able to change it. You have to decide to take responsibility for your thoughts, emotions, actions, and habits. We are going to look at some ways you can start taking back control of your thoughts and your life.

Psychology Today has an article entitled "Seeing Is Believing: The Power of Visualization" [Ref-10]. It says, "Brain studies now reveal that thoughts produce the same mental instructions as actions. Mental imagery impacts many cognitive processes in the brain: motor control, attention, perception, planning and memory. So the brain is getting trained for actual performance during visualization." It goes on to say, "Study results highlight the strength of the mind-body connection, or in other words the link between thoughts and behaviors – a very important connection for achieving your best life." The article also discusses how athletes use visualization in preparation for their competitions: "Seasoned athletes use vivid, highly detailed internal images and run-throughs of the entire performance, engaging all their senses in their mental rehearsal. . ."

Just like athletes, we can use visualization to achieve our goals in life. Ask anyone who has lost a lot of weight, and they will tell you that their mindset had everything to do with their success. Changing our mindset is not something that just happens. You have to consciously transform your thinking. I love the analogy of our mind being like the fertile soil in a garden. Our mind is where we plant our seeds of thought.

When planting a garden, you have to decide what it is that you want to grow. If you have a fresh patch of soil and do not make a decision about what to plant, weeds will begin to grow and eventually take over the entire patch. The same thing happens with our mind. If we do not make a decision of what we want in our lives, we become a victim of the circumstances in our life.

Let's say you decide to grow a beautiful daisy, but you plant a thistle seed. What is going to grow? The prickly thistle will sprout, of course, and not the beautiful daisy you wanted. This is the same with our mind as well. If we want to have lasting weight-loss success, we need to plant the seeds of success. However, if we plant the seed of failure, what is going to grow? Thoughts of failure. When failure grows in your mind, there is no room for success. Remember, what you focus on grows.

How do we plant the right seeds?

Weed out negative thinking. Self-talk can be our worst enemy when reaching toward our goals. Whenever you have a negative thought, stop immediately and replace it with the complete opposite, positive thought instead. For instance, if you are trying to do something new and think to yourself "I can't do this," stop immediately and replace that thought with "Yes, I will do this!"

Plant positive images of success. You need to have a vision of what the result is going to be. The more vivid the picture, the stronger it will be. Try to use as many of your senses as possible when developing your vision of success. What are you wearing, how do you feel, what are people saying to you, what do you see when you look in the mirror? Become emotionally attached to this new image of yourself. The picture you come up with should make you feel excited. You should get a great, big smile on your face whenever you think about it. If at any time your vision doesn't keep you excited, change it up so it becomes exciting again. This is crucial to making a new positive habit. Think about your vision as many times as possible during the day. At the very least, as soon as you wake up in the morning and before going to sleep at night. The more you think about your vision, the deeper the roots grow and the stronger it becomes. Create a vision board and keep it where you will see it often. You can cut photos out of magazines or download them from the internet and tape them to a poster board. Use photos that inspire you and keep your vision exciting. I have seen people put a picture of their head on the photo of the ideal body they want to have. That is strong reinforcement for your subconscious mind.

Pull out the weeds. Pesky garden weeds always grow and try to strangle the life out of our flowers. We must pull the weeds of negative thinking so they don't take root and overtake the exciting vision we have planted.

All gardens need to be watered. Every day you need to take an action that leads you closer to your vision. Daily, repeated and consistent behaviors create new habits.

You must tend to the garden of your mind every day. The seeds you plant will bloom. It is a law of nature, and we have all seen it work around us our entire lives. Make sure you plant the right seeds that lead you closer to your goal. Whatever you do, don't feed the weeds.

Another way to program our mind is with the use of affirmations. In the publication Society for Personality and Social Psychology [Ref-11], Sonia Kang, Ph.D. states, "Anytime you have low expectations for your performance, you tend to sink down and meet those low expectations, self-affirmation is a way to neutralize that threat." After having failed with so many diets, I certainly had low expectations when it came to losing weight. The repetitive use of affirmations helped me to break my pattern of negative thinking and habits. Once I started using affirmations consistently, my thoughts, emotions, and actions began to change.

As was mentioned earlier, the subconscious mind accepts whatever you tell it. Our subconscious does not have the reasoning ability that our conscious mind has. It doesn't differentiate between good or bad. The subconscious doesn't know the difference between what you perceive as truth versus the opposing facts. Our subconscious mind accepts whatever we have strong feelings about and works like a computer using an installed program. By using affirmations, we can begin to change the installed program by consciously changing our thinking.

We can target specific actions and feelings to help obtain the outcomes we want in our lives. With affirmations, you state a goal in a way that makes your subconscious mind believe the event has already taken place.

Here are three guidelines to use while setting up your new programming.

- Affirmations should always be spoken in a first person narrative. By using "I am" in front of your affirmation, the subconscious is more open to accepting the statement.
- Affirmations should always be stated in the present tense. By using words such as "I am" or "I know," your mind will believe the statement is already happening. Using statements like "I will" or "I think" allows doubt to creep into the subconscious mind.
- Affirmations should always be positive in nature. For example, the statement, "I am happy and healthy," is an affirmation. The statement, "I will try to be more happy and healthy," is not. "I eat healthy

food, every day," is an affirmation. "I'll start to eat healthy food every day," is not a correct affirmation.

You can also turn an affirmation into an empowering statement for yourself. When I worked with a life coach from Bob Proctor's organization, they gave me a card to carry around with my goal statement. It started out with, "I am so happy and grateful now that I ___." This is a great way to stay focused on your goal and reprogram your mind.

Here is an example of how you could use this:

"Today is (use a date 1 year from today), and I am so happy and grateful now that I am healthy, fit and weigh ___ pounds. I am worthy, deserving, powerful, capable, and confident." Whatever you use to complete the statement should make you feel excited about your future. Write it on an index card and carry it with you, use it as the wallpaper on your phone or computer. Tape it to the bathroom mirror. Put it wherever you are going to see it and read it. Dr Kang also says [Ref-11], "Writing down a self-affirmation may be more effective than just thinking it, but both methods can help." The key is repetition. The only way to reprogram your mind is through repetition. Get it? I'm using repetition on purpose to prove my point.

Repetition is what advertisers bombard us with all day long. They pay millions of dollars to program our minds. We have been subjected to their advertising our entire lives because repetition works. Instead of letting everyone else program our subconscious mind, it's time we started to program our own minds. Set the program for what you want to achieve.

Now you know how to start changing the program in your subconscious mind. Get started developing an exciting vision about your new life. Create a goal statement that you can read and say throughout the day. Remember that repetition is the key to setting yourself up for success. I like to repeat my statement at least five times in a row, three times a day: in the morning, at mid-day and then before falling asleep at night. The more often you repeat your statement, the faster you will see results. I have included a worksheet to help you develop your new mindset program on the next few pages. Use it to start setting your new program right away.

With Step 5 in the next chapter, I'm going to explain the "must have" ingredient for all success. Without this ingredient, positive results are impossible.

Goal Setting Worksheet

Step 1: Define Your Goal

_____

_____

_____

_____

_____

_____

_____

Gut check #1—Is my goal challenging but do-able?
Gut check #2 – Is my goal exciting enough to keep me focused every day?

Step 2: Define the Rewards for Achieving Your Goal

_____

_____

_____

_____

_____

_____

_____

What happens when you have achieved your goal?
List all the exciting ways your life will change.

Step 3: Write Your Goal Statement

I am so happy and grateful now that I am:

_____

_____

_____

_____

_____

_____

_____

_____

Write your goal as a positive statement with a date. You can use three months, six months or one year from today. (Example: It is June 25, 2017, and I am so happy and grateful that I weigh 140 lbs.)

Step 4: Break the Goal Down

What needs to be done MONTHLY to achieve my goal?

_____

_____

_____

_____

_____

_____

_____

What needs to be done WEEKLY to achieve my MONTHLY goals?

_____

_____

_____

_____

_____

_____

_____

_____

What needs be done DAILY to achieve my WEEKLY goals?

_____

_____

_____

_____

_____

_____

_____

_____

_____

_____

Step 5: Work the Plan

My schedule for working toward my goal is:

_____

_____

_____

_____

_____

_____

_____

_____

Step 6: Keep Your Goal in Front of Your Mind

This is where I will post my goal:

_____

_____

_____

_____

I will say my goal statement out loud at least three times per day at the following times:

_____

_____

_____

This is how I will document my progress:

_____

_____

_____

_____

_____

_____

_____

Choose a method that you will consistently work with to document your progress. It can be a simple paper journal or you can use an online app. It is important to track your progress daily. What you track gets done. It will give you the feedback to know if you are meeting your goals, or if a change to your plan is necessary.

Step 7:
Eliminate Subconscious Conflicts that May Impede Progress toward Your Goal

My positive affirmations are:

_____

_____

_____

_____

_____

Affirmation statements are positive and in the present tense. (Example: I am healthy, happy and fit.)

My big, exciting vision of how life will be after my goal is met:

_____

_____

_____

_____

_____

_____

_____

_____

_____

Write a detailed description of the perfect scene. Use as many of your physical senses that you can. It should be so exciting that it makes you smile whenever you think of it. You need to be emotionally charged by your vision. Use a separate sheet of paper if needed.

My first positive action in the direction of my goal is:

_____

_____

_____

_____

_____

_____

_____

CHAPTER FIVE

LIGHTS, CAMERA, ACTION

*The difference between who you are and
who you want to be is what you do.*
Bill Phillips

Now that you know how to train your brain, it's time to start taking steps toward your new healthy lifestyle. Just like filming a big Hollywood movie, if there is no "Action," the film would never be made. The same goes for how we live our lives. We may know what to do and that we need to do it, we may have even started to train our brain, but without taking "Action," nothing will get done.

Cary Grant, star of many Hollywood classic films, said, "I began by acting like the person I wanted to be, and eventually I became that person" [Ref-12]. We can all learn from that. Much like an actor, we can begin to act like a healthy, fit person long enough to actually become a healthy, fit person. Whether you feel ready or not, start to act the part of who you want to be. You will develop the mindset of that type of person, and eventually you will become that person.

For months after my surgery, I didn't feel healthy and definitely not fit. I was still in need of using a wheelchair for at least six months after surgery. It wasn't until I lost 150 pounds that I started to see and feel a difference in being able to walk and breathe at the same time. Even though I didn't feel healthy and fit, in my mind I was acting healthy and fit. I could see that the weight was dropping, and I was shrinking out of my clothes. I had faith that I would soon feel healthy and fit, too.

I began to act the part of the person I was hoping to become. I began shopping for fitness equipment even though there was no way I could exercise yet. I visualized myself taking long bike rides along the lake front. I made a list of all the activities I was going to do the next summer. Then one night when I was out to dinner with friends, I realized I was eating dinner like a healthy, fit person. It was another light bulb moment. I was eating like a "normal" person. How could I eat like a normal person? I was never a normal person when it came to food.

It doesn't matter how you feel at this exact moment. You must start to take an action toward your new healthy lifestyle. The tennis legend Arthur Ashe said, "Start where you are. Use what you have. Do what you can." There is no waiting for tomorrow, Monday, next month or the New Year. If you truly want to change, you must take an action immediately. That is the difference between the person who succeeds and the person who does not.

Notice I did not say to change every action you take immediately. I said take "an action," one action immediately. That is how we start the process of change, one step at a time. If you feel like you are ready to take a giant step, go right ahead, but I know to begin the process of change, it was easier for me to take one step at a time. It is much easier to make a small change in your behavior and continue to build from there, one success at a time. Trying to start out too big can be overwhelming and cause us to quit before we even get started. This is especially true for those of us who haven't seen a success for a while. I have included a Personal Action Worksheet at the end of this chapter. It can help you decide what action to start with if you are unsure where to begin.

By starting with small action steps and succeeding, we are able to build our confidence. When we build our confidence, we can begin to accomplish bigger actions. This is a principle known as momentum, and it is a powerful force. Once you begin the process of working toward a goal, you do not stop until it's achieved. Say this out loud: "I will not stop until my goal is achieved." That is worth repeating again.

Ever been on a plane or watch one speed down the runway? It starts slowly taxiing to the runway. Then, with all the power it has, it starts speeding faster and faster, until it lifts off the ground and climbs into the sky. It is amazing to see. The same principle that lifts those behemoth objects into the sky applies to us in our everyday lives.

Think about how you may have used momentum without even realizing it. For a lot of us, the first sign of momentum was thinking about having bariatric surgery. Then we went to a seminar, saw a doctor, the nutritionist, a psychologist, special testing, insurance approval, and who knows what else, just to schedule the surgery. These are probably some of the biggest hurdles we ever had to jump through. Or maybe some of you are going through this right now.

Since you are reading this book, I'm pretty sure you didn't quit at the first uncomfortable situation. You were bound and determined to get your surgery and worked every day until you got there. Welcome to the force of momentum.

If at any point you decided it wasn't worth the effort and quit, you would still be in the same old situation you were in before. That is why we cannot quit. Once we have started to take action, we must continue with the momentum until we reach our goal. That's not to say that perfection is expected. Just don't quit until you have reached your goal. It is reported in the *European Journal of Social Psychology* [Ref-13] that researchers from the University College London, UK [Ref-14] did a study about habit formation. They found that participants in their study did not have a noticeable difference to their habit formation when they missed a day of their new routine. However, if they missed a week, there was a noticeable negative effect on that habit's formation.

When a setback occurs, pick yourself up right away, just like the old saying, "Get back on the horse." When I was younger, I fell off a couple horses. The first time, I was so afraid to try again that it took years to get back on one. The second time, I got right back on the horse and was able to enjoy many more wonderful rides. I lost years of enjoying my love for horses because I lacked the courage to try again. When you have a setback, don't wait a week beating yourself up for a negative behavior. Pick back up where you left off and move forward again. If you have been taking one step at a time, it is easy to begin again. You don't have to start from scratch; you just continue building from where you left off.

Speaking of setbacks, there is another part of our nature that affects the way we look at certain actions. Some actions cause a strong emotional response with us. When that emotion is positive, we will do that action often and consistently. If the emotion is negative, we may try to do that action for awhile, but we usually end up quitting after a short time or we may not even try at all.

When you start to take on a new action step, create a positive affirmation to train your brain for the new behavior. Create an affirmation that will re-enforce the positive emotions needed for the consistent development of the new behavior. Visualize the benefits you will see and feel for having consistently taken that new action toward your goal. What great rewards await you for taking this new action consistently?

Now you know the most important ingredient to seeing results. You must take action if you want to improve your life. Use the Personal Action Worksheet at the end of this chapter to help you choose an important action to start with.

In the next chapter with Step 6, we will see how to use your actions to create an easy and natural flow to your new healthy and fit lifestyle.

Personal Action Worksheet

What is one thing you could do (but are not doing now) on a regular basis that would make an important, positive difference in your life?

_____

_____

_____

_____

_____

_____

_____

_____

_____

Why aren't you doing it regularly?

_____

_____

_____

_____

_____

_____

_____

_____

What can you do, right now, to incorporate this into your life consistently? How would you feel doing this regularly?

_____

_____

_____

_____

_____

_____

_____

_____

Record the date, time and how you feel when you complete this action for the next seven days.

_____

_____

_____

_____

_____

_____

_____

_____

CHAPTER SIX

HABITUAL BEHAVIORS

Success is the sum of small efforts, repeated day in and day out.
Robert Collier

Now you know the importance of taking "action" every day toward your goal. Let's begin to use those actions to create your new healthy habits. Long-term success on our bariatric journey comes down to the "habits we keep" and the "habits we create."

One of my all-time favorite quotes since having bariatric surgery is from Socrates: "The secret of change is to focus all of your energy, not on fighting the old, but on building the new." Reading this was really another light bulb moment. It made perfect sense for what I was feeling about this journey.

Most of my life was spent fighting old habits when it came to losing weight. Whenever I tried to diet, I felt deprived. Negative thoughts ran through my head all day long. *Why can't I eat like everyone else? Look at what they are eating! It's not fair that I gain weight so easily. I can't do this. Nothing ever works.*

Then I would start to call myself names I would never call anyone else. Awful names like fat pig, disgusting loser and blob. I was one big ball of negative energy. I used the "momentum principle" pretty darn good, but it was in the wrong direction.

Those same old thoughts crept in when I came home after having my Sleeve Surgery. The food, oh, how I missed the food. I knew the rest of the world was out there eating like they always had, but I wasn't able to anymore. Even though I had worked so hard and long to have weight-loss surgery, those thoughts rushed in like a flood. Ever hear that old saying, "Wherever you go, there you are"? No matter how hard I tried, I found myself fighting those same old thoughts.

After reading the Socrates quote, I made a conscious decision to change the way I was looking at my situation. I decided to stop fighting my old thoughts and behaviors and to embrace a new way of thinking. I stopped thinking about what I was missing and began to think about everything I was gaining with this new lifestyle. I was getting pieces of my life back every day. It seems miraculous now; the struggle finally stopped. I was free from the thoughts and feelings I had held onto for so long. It was like stepping out of a shadow that I had purposely kept with me. I gave myself permission to become the new person I was supposed to be. I was done keeping myself in a little box on the shelf, waiting for the perfect time to open it.

In his book *The Greatest Salesman in the World*, Og Mandino wrote: ". . .the only difference between those who have failed and those who have succeeded lies in the differences of their habits. Good habits are the key to all success. Bad habits are the unlocked door to failure" [Ref-15]. Later he goes on to say, "For it is another of nature's laws that only a habit can subdue another habit" [Ref-16].

The easiest way to let go of an old negative habit is to replace it with a new positive habit. You don't just stop an old habit; you REPLACE that habit with a NEW habit. I'm repeating this for a reason. I had read Og Mandino's book a few times and never realized the true meaning of "only a habit can subdue another habit." It wasn't until after reading the Socrates quote, "The secret of change is to focus all of your energy, not on fighting the old, but on building the new" that I finally understood what I needed to do.

In an article at HopesandFears.com, Elliot Berkman Ph.D [Ref-17], a neuroscientist, confirmed what I finally had realized. He states, "It's much easier to start doing something new than to stop doing something habitual without a replacement behavior."

I began to "build" my new life. All of my energy, focus and determination went to building the new me and not on fighting what I used to be. Talk about freedom! If I was going to be consumed by any habit, it would now be a new positive, healthy habit.

I began with changing the routines I had around food. No more mindlessly scarfing my food down. If I couldn't eat as much as I had before, I was going to be conscious and mindful of what I was able to eat. That meant I no longer ate in front of the TV, computer, tablet, phone or a book. I sat down at a table with my food and enjoyed each precious bite. I enjoyed the texture, the taste and appearance of each savory nibble. If I had a craving for something sweet, I ate a piece of fruit. If I wanted something crunchy, I ate a slice of a peeled cucumber. I satisfied the cravings with a new healthy alternative and that became my new healthy habit.

Just yesterday I was given the option to eat cherry licorice but preferred to have an actual cherry instead. Did I feel deprived? Absolutely NOT. My new positive habits have been ingrained into my new mindset. I don't miss the old behaviors or the way they made me feel. My new habits have given me my life and future back. That's a whole lot better!

The important thing to keep in mind when building your new healthy lifestyle is that habits only become habits through repetition. When you repeat the behavior over and over again, you create a habit. As we learned in the previous chapter, you must use the "momentum principle" to create your new healthy habit. Every time you go back to an old, negative habit, you lose ground with the new habit and strengthen the old habit once again.

The new routines you create can be in every area of your life, not just for meals. After I stopped eating in front of the TV, I realized I didn't enjoy TV at other times of the day either. I started a new hobby and began writing. This activity was much more enjoyable and productive. Plus, it had no connection to any of my old food behaviors. I eventually created a whole new way of life that had nothing at all to do with any of my old food patterns.

When creating your new habits, it is important to know your impulse foods. By being aware of your impulse foods, you can avoid the circumstances that might lead you into a vulnerable state. Plan ahead and have replacement options available to keep you on course. You never know when a sneaky food temptation might show up.

One of my more memorable temptations showed up while I was at the emergency room one very late night. Somehow I ended up in the waiting room seated right in front of the vending machines. There was this lovely, little, yellow package staring at me, winking at me. It was Peanut M&Ms. We had a long history together, sort of like childhood sweethearts. This was one of those stressful times when the "ever so helpful M&M" just wanted to comfort me and soothe my nerves. I'm not sure how long I sat there staring at that thoughtful M&M wooing me through the glass. I just hope it wasn't obvious to everyone else in the room. I eventually told the M&M I wasn't that kind of girl anymore. I appreciated its concern, but I just wouldn't feel right about a one night stand. I used humor to deflect the advance of an unhealthy behavior, and it worked.

Include your family members and friends in your new healthy routines. That will make it easier for you and healthier for them. If going out with friends and having beer and pizza on a Friday night was your fun night, make plans to do something different that doesn't revolve around food. Don't deprive yourself of friends; just create a new way of enjoying those friendships.

Creating a new habit requires a concentrated effort in the beginning, but the results are worth the effort. By taking the actions that lead you to success today, you will be liberated for the rest of your life. Haven't you already served the penalty for your old habits? Effort is required for both good and bad habits. Choose the effort that will make the rest of your life the best part of your life.

Now you know how habits can be changed to empower your life. Let's move on to Step 7: The Secret Sauce of Success.

CHAPTER SEVEN

THE SECRET SAUCE OF SUCCESS

Have patience. All things are difficult before they become easy.
Saadi

Now you know the foundation blocks of making a lasting change in your life. It's time to learn Step 7, what I call the Secret Sauce of Success. This special sauce has three ingredients: Patience, Persistence, and Perseverance.

Our bariatric journey is filled with emotional ups and downs. It often takes longer to arrive at our destination than we originally thought. In those moments of frustration, we decide our fate. Should we keep going, or is it futile to continue?

Anyone who has ever had bariatric surgery will tell you the surgery is not the easy way out. People who have had success will tell you that it's the best decision they have ever made, and yet there are those who say their surgery failed because they gained some or all of their weight back.

I knew all of that when I started my journey to become healthy again. My dad had weight-loss surgery in 1986. Bariatric surgery was in the dark ages back then. He was cut from his chest to his abdomen and suffered too many complications to list. He went back and forth to the hospital for months and felt sick most of that time. But he did start to lose weight, which was his goal. I watched as he happily lost 150 pounds only to gain most of it back again. He had no idea that his surgery was a tool and not a lifetime fix.

Bariatric surgery is not a "magic pill." Maintaining weight loss will take consistent effort for the rest of our lives. If at any point we allow old, unhealthy habits back into our routines, we will experience weight gain. That is pretty much guaranteed. Do we need to be perfect? Absolutely not, but we need to be at least ninety percent effective.

I'm going to say this again: What we do often and consistently will become a habit. Knowing this to be a fundamental truth, I made the decision not to eat certain "impulse" foods ever again. Just like a recovering alcoholic knows they cannot ever drink again, I know there are certain foods I can't risk ever eating again. Knowing this has not made my life less enjoyable; in fact, it has given me more opportunities. Being patient, persistent and using perseverance has given me a life back to live.

Like the quote at the beginning of this chapter says, patience is required. Patience is your ability to accept delays. Patience is knowing that some things take time to accomplish. You have to stay with your new healthy behaviors until they become your new habits. Once a behavior becomes a habit, this will be your natural and automatic way of dealing with food. You won't even think about it anymore.

As mentioned in an earlier chapter, researchers from the University College London conducted a study [Ref-14] regarding habit formation in 2009. They found an average of 66 days was required by their participants to develop a new habit. Individual times required from the participants ranged from 18 days to 254 days. They also found that participants took longer to create an exercise habit than it did to change an eating behavior. It takes time to change our behaviors, but it definitely can be done.

As Saadi said, "All things are difficult before they become easy." You have seen this principle work your entire life. Ever wonder what would happen if a toddler thought like an adult does? What if they fell down twice while learning to walk and said, "Forget it, I can't do this. I'll just crawl around the floor for the rest of my life." Thankfully, that doesn't happen. They keep getting back up and trying until they can walk all by themselves. What about learning to ride a bike or drive a car? None of it was easy in the beginning, but the more we did those activities the easier it became. The actions to balance ourselves while we walked or rode our bikes became a natural habit, and we just started doing them without thinking. That was the point at which the activity became easy for us.

Persistence, our second ingredient, is defined by the The Merriam Webster Dictionary [Ref-17b] as "the quality that allows someone to continue doing something or trying to do something even though it is difficult . . ." That is why I absolutely love this quote from Paramahansa Yogananda. It opened my mind and literally changed my perceptions during my weight-loss journey: "Persistence guarantees that results are inevitable." Read that again, slowly. Here is another quote from Og Mandino's book, *The Greatest Salesman in the World* [Ref-18]: "So long as there is breath in me, that long will I persist. For now I know one of the greatest principles of success; if I persist long enough I will win." As long as we persist with our healthy behaviors, we will see success. It is as simple as that. No question about it. Persist with the healthy actions until they become new habits. Persist with the healthy habits, and you will reach your goal. Continue to persist with the healthy habits, and you can have lifelong weight-loss success.

Which brings us to perseverance. As we persist with our healthy behaviors, perseverance is what keeps us going no matter what else gets in the way. TheFreeDictionary.com [Ref-18b] defines perseverance as "continued steady belief or efforts, withstanding discouragement or difficulty . . ." Yes, there will be obstacles, challenges and discouraging moments on our journey. However, it is important not to allow those issues to get in the way of our goals. When we persevere, we look around the obstacles, challenges and discouragement for solutions. We don't get sidetracked or quit. We keep moving forward, knowing that we will reach our goals, and perseverance is what will allow us to maintain our goal for the rest of our lives.

I kind of laugh when I think about my first experience hitting a weight-loss stall after surgery. In the past when I hit a stall, I would get discouraged and start eating everything I had given up during the diet. About six weeks after surgery, I experienced my first stall. I wanted to eat everything I hadn't eaten for weeks, but at that point in time, it was physically impossible to eat any of those foods. I was discouraged on many levels, but as you read in the previous chapters, I eventually found ways to deal with the situations as they arose. I also found out that hitting weight-loss stalls would be a common occurrence during my journey. You hit quite a few stalls when you lose 224 pounds. The good news was that every stall ended. And weight-loss would continue again: there was a distinct pattern.

When you use the "secret sauce" of patience, persistence and perseverance, you know that no matter what is happening around you, success will be inevitable. You must truly believe success is inevitable. When you believe that without a doubt, nothing will stop you from reaching your goal. In the next chapter we will cover Step 8, the most talked about characteristic of successful people.

CHAPTER EIGHT

THE POWER OF YOUR THOUGHTS

*You must learn a new way to think
before you can master a new way to be.*
Marianne Williamson

You now have all but one of the ingredients that allowed me to change my old behaviors and mindset. Finally, and just as important is Step 8, a positive mindset. Positive thinking has gotten a bad rap from some people. However, positive thinking is necessary for making changes in our lives. I have saved this topic for last because it's the glue that keeps everything else together.

Positive thinking by itself will not change your life. But positive thinking along with taking positive actions will change your life. It was reported at NCBI.NLM.NIH.gov [Ref-18c] in 2013 that researchers from the University of North Carolina found ". . . one group of individuals began a mind-training practice that increased their positive emotions and, in turn, their personal resources and well-being." It went on to say, "When people open their hearts to positive emotions, they seed their own growth in ways that transform them for the better."

I came head to head with my negative thinking before my decision to have bariatric surgery. The root of my weight-loss failures were my negative attitude and self-critical thinking. Then my weight-loss failures turned into the failure in almost everything I attempted to do. I was watching my life slip away, piece by piece. I weighed 394 pounds, lost my business, was in a wheelchair and had trouble breathing. I felt like a big blob that could no longer function. I had surrendered and was no longer in control of my life. Needless to say, that was the lowest point of my existence. Looking back now, I don't even know how I made it through the surgery approval process.

Positive thinking is more than just a Pollyanna saying. It's about expecting positive things in your life. What you expect has a pretty funny way of showing up in your life. When you expect great things, your whole world begins to change. You stop looking for the reasons why something can't work, and you start to look for ways to make it work. You don't look for excuses to not do something; you find the way to do it.

When you think you cannot do something, you will not be able to do it. How can you do anything that you don't believe can be done? It's as simple as that. So, yes, we do need to think positive and believe that we can accomplish what we set out to do. When I dieted in the past, I always felt deprived, but I used my willpower to eat right and exercise. I was just waiting for the moment I could go back to my normal behaviors again. We all know how that works.

Believing in yourself is one of the biggest ways to remove the roadblocks you have to your long-term success. You must know that this time your tool has given you an advantage you never had before. This time is different. This time you can definitely lose the weight once and for all. But you need to know this at your very core. Every fiber of your being must know that you can and will do this. Be like the beautiful butterfly that doesn't go back into its cocoon. Decide today that the new you has emerged and refuse to ever let the old behaviors back into your life.

Knowing whether you are having positive or negative thoughts seems like a simple process, but in the beginning you must make a conscious effort to check your thinking. You have been thinking a certain way your entire life. Now you need to pay attention to your thinking and choose to create positive thoughts. That will give you the opportunity to begin the process of changing your expectations, behavior and actions.

Here is a great way to know what kind of thoughts you are thinking. Pay attention to your emotions and your feelings. When you are thinking in a positive way, you feel happy and excited about life. When you are thinking in a negative way, there is an opposite effect. You feel sad, depressed and look for the negative in everything around you. When you realize your emotions are low, stop immediately and change the way you are thinking. You cannot think a positive and negative thought at the same time. Replace the negative thought with the complete opposite, positive thought. That is the fastest and simplest way to switch your thought patterns. Sometimes it can help to say "Stop" out loud to break the pattern when switching your thoughts. If you are out in a crowded area, you might get some looks. But then again, maybe not. Just pretend you are on your cell phone. You may also want to keep a log to record your thoughts and emotions throughout the day. With a written record available, you will be able to see if there are patterns to your feelings or certain triggers that affect your emotions. When you are aware of patterns and triggers, you can make a course correction sooner.

Sometimes, I still have thoughts about missing my favorite food or beverage from the old days. When I do, I immediately change that thought to how great my life has been without that particular item. I focus on the results I'm seeing and how great I feel compared to how I felt when I used to indulge that behavior. I literally look at the situation as the "old me" versus the "new me." The "new me" is so much stronger than the "old me" ever was. The same will be true for you.

Another way negative thoughts influence us is through our environment. When you start to make changes in your life, it's important to give yourself an advantage. By controlling your environment, you can stop the negativity from entering into your life. Your environment is constantly bombarded by outside influences. The media and people around you have a bigger impact on your thinking than you might realize. Do yourself a favor and set yourself up for success.

Here are a few steps I took to change my environment and take back control of my life.

- I started by changing what I watched and read. That old statement, "Garbage In, Garbage Out," is true. I was a news junky for years. Constantly watching, reading and listening to the news every chance I got. It made me angry all the time. How could I expect to feel positive about anything when I filled my mind with negativity every day? Instead, I began to spend my time reading positive and inspiring books. I began researching new, exciting goals and feeling grateful for all the good in my life.
- I distanced myself from negative people and would remove myself from negative conversations. The difference was like night and day. Negative people are a drag to be around. They want everyone to feel as bad as they do, just like that old saying, "Misery loves company."
- I began to focus on my lifelong dreams. I started to keep a list of the all the things I wanted to do. The list included everything I thought I would never be able to do when I weighed 394 pounds. I started to

take action and began doing the things on my list. At first, this process was slow because I had a lot of weight to lose. As I started to do these things, however, my list grew to even bigger dreams and goals. It's now an ongoing process that keeps me excited about life.

Always focus on the expansion and freedom to live your life in a new and empowering way. Don't focus on what you are lacking or missing. Be grateful for where you are today because you know that tomorrow will be even better. Expect great things to happen, and you will see great things in your life.

CONCLUSION

Permanent results come from permanent changes...
Joel Fuhrman

Now you know the steps necessary to make a lasting change with your old food behaviors. Remember that this is not a diet. This is a way of life. Look at bariatric surgery as a tool to help you achieve and maintain your goal. That means you need to use the tool correctly today, tomorrow, the next day and the next. If we gain weight back, it's not that our surgery failed us; it's more like we failed our surgery (except in cases of medical complications).

In her book *Eat It Up*, psychologist Connie Stapleton Ph.D. tells the story of a patient, a man who asked his surgeon if it was okay to eat hot dogs. His surgeon replied, yes, it was okay to eat hot dogs. So, the young man started to eat hot dogs again. Dr. Stapleton explained to the man, ". . . just because you can physically digest a hot dog, doesn't mean it is a good choice for you" [Ref-19]. That reminds me of some of the comments I hear from people who have gained weight back after surgery. They explain that they need a surgery revision because they can eat a whole lot more food now than they could right after surgery. Just like Dr. Stapleton said, just because you can eat a whole lot more doesn't mean you should. That is why changing our thoughts and behaviors about food is so important. Lasting weight-loss occurs when we make lasting changes to our behaviors.

It is important to keep moving forward with your life. There is no such thing as standing still in your success. You either move forward or you go backwards. Make the decision right now that your life will be one of forward movement. When you reach a goal, set a new exciting goal. Do not become complacent and revert back to old behaviors. Use these principles to stay in control of your thoughts and your life.

The eight steps you have just learned are the exact steps that allowed me to change my old food behaviors and my entire life. I spent years studying these principles. Then, after my surgery, all the pieces finally fit together like a puzzle. These principles will work in every area of your life to achieve what is important to you.

Let's review what you have learned.
- You know to accept your past but not let it define your future.
- Now you know what to do by following the Bariatric Basics.
- You will do what you know because you learned how your mind works and what is needed to think differently.
- You can train your brain by focusing on your success using visualization and affirmations.

- You know how important it is to take action every day toward your vision.
- You have the information to change your habits from unhealthy behaviors to new healthy behaviors.
- You know the importance of being patient, persistent and to persevere through all obstacles.
- The glue that holds everything together is positive thinking.

Here are a few more lessons I have learned during my journey so far.

- Don't demand perfection. Trying to be perfect sets us up to fail. When a mistake is made, learn from it and move on. Think about making progress, not about being perfect.
- Let go of the hurt and pain from the past. We can only move forward by releasing the negative thoughts and feelings that have held us back for way too long.
- Build your confidence. Take small steps in the beginning, and build to bigger steps. The small victories will turn into larger ones. With each victory, your confidence grows.
- Be true to yourself. Don't let anyone or anything sway you from living the life you deserve.
- Be kind to yourself. Stop self-critical thinking and replace it with positive affirmations.
- Don't invite temptation into your life by trying an impulse food or beverage. It's just not worth it.

- Failure is feedback. I don't believe in failure anymore. I lived with it for too long. There is no room for failure in my new life. When things don't go as planned, I see that as feedback. I just find out what doesn't work, I learn from it and move forward. That makes life much more rewarding.

- Don't compare yourself to others. Comparing ourselves to others takes away the joy we have with our own progress. Everyone's journey is different. If others have difficulties, it does not mean you will. If others lose weight faster, it doesn't mean you are slow. "A flower does not think of competing to the flower next to it. It just blooms," writes Zen Shin. Appreciate where YOU are today and believe in yourself. Your life is special and unique. Celebrate being YOU!

In this book I have given you the steps to take control of your thinking and your life. They are simple to implement, and they work. Now it is your turn. Take action and use these principles in your life. Take the time, right now, to apply what you have read and create your own personal Mindset Breakthrough. Be like the caterpillar that transforms into a beautiful butterfly with wings and soars to new heights. Break through your barriers and begin to experience life without limits. Change starts the moment you take that very first step.

Before we end our time together, I would like to invite you to join my motivational community. It's easy to do using your phone. Just text **LIVING** to **444999.**

Know that you are not alone. Know that there is hope, and never give up. This is not an easy path. But it can be one of the most amazing journeys of your life.

I'm gonna make the rest of my life the best of my life.
Unknown

BIBLIOGRAPHY

[Ref- 1]
http://www.riversideonline.com/employees/myhealthylife
style/newsletter/half-hour-window.cfm?RenderForPrint=1
[Ref– 2]
http://bariatrics.ucla.edu/workfiles/UCLA-Bariatric-posto
perative-diet-instructions.pdf
[Ref- 3]
http://www.hopkinsmedicine.org/johns_hopkins_bayview
/_docs/medical_services/bariatrics/nutrition_weight_loss
_surgery.pdf
[Ref- 4]
http://www.bariatric-surgery-source.com/bariatric-diet.ht
ml#4._Drink
[Ref- 5]
http://www.heart.org/HEARTORG/HealthyLiving/Physi
calActivity/FitnessBasics/American-Heart-Association-Rec
ommendations-for-Physical-Activity-in-Adults_UCM_3079
76_Article.jsp#.V_RDJPkrJdi
[Ref- 6]
http://www.obesitycoverage.com/gastric-sleeve-reference-
manual/
[Ref- 7]
http://www.everydayhealth.com/weight/busting-the-musc
le-weighs-more-than-fat-myth.aspx
[Ref- 8]
https://asmbs.org/patients/life-after-bariatric-surgery

[Ref- 9]
http://toosmall.org/news/commentaries/childs-first-5-yea
rs-hold-key-to-success
[Ref-10]
https://www.psychologytoday.com/blog/flourish/200912
/seeing-is-believing-the-power-visualization
[Ref-11]
http://www.spsp.org/news-center/press-releases/self-affir
mations-may-calm-jitters-and-boost-performance-research-
finds
[Ref-12]
https://www.goodreads.com/author/quotes/74344.Cary_
Grant
[Ref-13]
http://onlinelibrary.wiley.com/doi/10.1002/ejsp.674/abst
ract
[Ref-14]
https://www.ucl.ac.uk/news/news-articles/0908/0908040
1
[Ref-15] Mandino, O. 1974 *The Greatest Salesman in the World*, USA Bantam, P 54
[Ref-16] Mandino, O. 1974 *The Greatest Salesman in the World*, USA Bantam, P 55
[Ref-17]
http://www.hopesandfears.com/hopes/now/question/21
6479-how-long-does-it-really-take-to-break-a-habit
[Ref-17b]
http://www.merriam-webster.com/dictionary/persistence
[Ref-18] Mandino, O. 1974 *The Greatest Salesman in the World*, USA Bantam, P 67

[Ref-18b] http://www.thefreedictionary.com/perseverance
[Ref-18c]
https://www.ncbi.nlm.nih.gov/pmc/articles/PMC315602
8/
[Ref-19] Stapleton, C 2009 *Eat It Up!: The Complete
Mind/Body/Spirit Guide to a Full Life After Weight Loss Surgery*,
USA Mind Body Health Services, Inc, P 104

ABOUT THE AUTHOR

Beth Bianca is a bariatric patient who lost 224 pounds. She is the founder of LadiesInWeighting.com and a contributing author to the Huffington Post.

After weighing 394 pounds and riddled with health issues, Beth received a second chance at life by having weight-loss surgery. She is passionate about sharing the lessons she has learned and providing support to other bariatric patients.

Beth is a Certified Life Coach and Lifestyle & Weight Management Specialist. You can find her at LadiesInWeighting.com and connect with her on Facebook.

Made in the USA
Lexington, KY
06 October 2017